CHOOSING DIABETES

KELLEY AKINS

INDIGORIVER
PUBLISHING

CHOOSING DIABETES

Editors: Christian Pacheco, Donna Melillo

Cover Photography: Rhonda Harper Photography/ rhondaharperphotography.com

Cover Design: Jason Kauffmann / Firelight Interactive / firelightinteractive.com

Interior Design: Kevin Williamson/kevinwilliamsondesign.com

Indigo River Publishing
3 West Garden Street Ste. 352
Pensacola, FL 32502
www.indigoriverpublishing.com

Ordering Information:
Quantity sales: Special discounts are available on quantity purchases by corporations, associations, and others. For details, contact the publisher at the address above.

Orders by U.S. trade bookstores and wholesalers: Please contact the publisher at the address above.

Printed in the United States of America

Library of Congress Control Number: 2016931449

ISBN: 978-0-9962330-8-8

First Edition

With Indigo River Publishing, you can always expect great books, strong voices, and meaningful messages. Most importantly, you'll always find ... words worth reading.

To Mom and Dad, who
when they got the call
left the mower running
and the pot boiling over
to come to me. You are
why I never give up.

About the Author

Kelley Akins, MS, LPCi is a Type 1 Diabetic that lives and works in Dallas, TX. Receiving her diagnosis in 2009 gave the push she needed to begin to accomplish certain lifelong goals set for herself but hadn't yet achieved. For instance, she received her master's degree in 2013 from Southern Methodist University and traveled abroad to Israel. During her time at SMU, she ran a support group for diabetics and was able to participate in some of the local JDRF functions which allowed her feel connected to the diabetic community.

Initially, the lack of emotional support she experienced at the time of her diagnosis led her to want to help others that found themselves in a similar situation. She understands firsthand the challenges of receiving a diagnosis, searching for a physician and reaching for support that does not seem readily available. Being diabetic and a counselor places her in the unique position, having both the personal experience with what it feels like to manage diabetes on a daily basis and the credentials to guide others to a more positive mindset with which to manage their own. She is dedicated to bringing awareness to how important emotional health is to good diabetes management.

Kelley enjoys a close relationship with her friends and family. She enjoys traveling and is an avid reader. She has a four-pound Chihuahua named Bubbles that has been her sidekick for 11 years. She prides herself on being an aunt to her own family and several surrogate families and cherishes her long term friendships.

Acknowledgements

would like to acknowledge that I had no idea when I started this it would become something that would be in the hands of other diabetics and would actually be helping people. I sometimes journal an experience so that the details are not lost with the passing of time. This is how it all started and was definitely one of the activities that got me through. I would like to thank John Bradshaw for coming to SMU, giving me the inspiration, and putting me on the path. I would also like to thank Dr. Anthony Picchioni for always encouraging me and giving me much needed guidance. I deeply respect you and the education I received at Southern Methodist University. I would like to thank Tom Hartsell for his professional assistance and also pointing me in the right direction.

I want to thank my mom for proofing what I wrote when the idea of making this into a book began to form.

Thank you for always giving it to me straight with love and encouragement...no words can ever explain how much I know you and Dad love me. Thank you for eternally dropping everything for me! I want to say thank you to my pals Dr. Carolyn Greenleaf and Kellie King for being my cheerleaders. Thanks to Jeff Casey for a lifetime of friendship and laughing at myself and for your unwavering support. Thank you to Emily, who replays my youth right in front of me and sometimes lets me go back to that moment of splendor in the grass with her! To all the J's in my life—please let this inspire you. Thank you to my best friend April Peterson for loving me through everything I've thrown at her. Thank you to my brothers, Jody and Paul, for a lifetime of love and laughter. I appreciate all of the family and friends who have encouraged me through my diagnosis and along this path. I couldn't make it without you! I especially want to thank everyone at Indigo River Publishing. I'm spoiled forever.

Foreword

A year and half ago, I came out of a 23-day hospitalization for congestive heart failure brought on by Chronic Obstruction Pulmonary Disorder (COPD). The powerful steroids that were administered to me during my hospital stay created a drug-induced early diabetes. It is a great coincidence that Kelley Akins, a bright and creative graduate student I taught at SMU, had sent me the book *Choosing Diabetes*, which I had encouraged her to write. I never realized she would be helping me manage my newly diagnosed disease—Kelley's personal experience and her exceptional emotional intelligence give her the ability to write cogently about the emotional aspects of diabetes.

Choosing Diabetes is a much-needed help for people dealing with and emotionally managing the disease of diabetes. She is taking diabetes out of the closet, so to speak, and reducing the anxiety, bewilderment, and often downright shame that surrounds it. Realizing the stigma and shame she felt when diagnosed with Type 1 diabetes at age 39, Kelley figured out that the facts of the disease were not as devastating as the emotional fantasies that come with it. She has used the wisdom of the Greek philosopher Epictetus, who clearly saw that what happens in a person's life ultimately depends on the way a person thinks and feels about what happened. Or as Don Juan, the sorcerer Carlos Castenda writes about, says, "We either make ourselves miserable, or we make ourselves strong. The amount of work is the same." Managing and positively thinking about your diabetes is critical—how we label and interpret things is our choice.

Kelley Akins offers us a step-by-step and almost day-by-day way of finding a livable and comfortable way to deal with our disease. This helps us to cope with the mostly well-meaning but ignorant things people ask us about it. In fact, this book can help you learn how to support and nourish your diabetic friends and loved ones.

I found Kelley's book especially valuable for friends and family members of a person with diabetes. The most important thing I got out of reading Kelley's book was her focus on living in the now and taking one day at a time. I have long lived by the poem that has guided millions of alcoholics to stability and sobriety:

Look to this day for it is life
The very life of life—
For every yesterday is
but a dream
And every tomorrow a vision—
And today well lived, makes
every yesterday a dream of
happiness
And every tomorrow a vision
of hope!

Kelley tells us that the physical management of Type 1 diabetes takes only about 15 minutes a day—Type 2, even less. Don't surrender your one and only life to a few minutes a day. Carpe Diem!

John Bradshaw Author of three #1 New York Times Bestselling Books and voted by colleagues and peers as one of the most important writers on emotional health in the 20th century.

Preface

Diabetes is largely misunderstood by most people. So when the diagnosis comes knocking at your door, it's a scary thing. I applaud you for having the courage to understand something that shocks, confuses, or frightens you. That alone proves you are stronger in this very moment than you think you are. You may not believe this, but diabetes could quite possibly be the best thing that ever happened to you. My diabetes is a mirror I can peer into at any given time that will tell me exactly how I am treating myself. It will be your friend, or it will be your worst enemy. The best part is that you decide which one it is.

In the first few hours, the first few weeks, and then the first few months, you are getting to know your disease. Life is a negotiation, and this is no different. I am not saying there will be no unpleasant moments—nothing is a complete bed of roses. But you can reduce the impact of this by making the right choices—the choices you probably have put off making for far too long. Eat, exercise, rest, sleep, peace. If you think you are too busy for diabetes, it will do its damage silently, so as not to bother you.

But this is not another book about a medical condition. It is a way of perceiving and accepting a disease that you are now past having a choice about. My advice is to not indulge yourself for very long with "Why me?" Just stay open to getting to know diabetes and, more importantly, getting to know yourself. In the beginning, friends and family would give me a very sad face and say, "I'm so sorry." Even now in my day-to-day life, people will do the same. Whether I share my personal story with them or not, the feeling I have is always the same: don't waste one second feeling sorry for me. Diabetes saved my life and paved the way for a whole new one. I got clear with what I wanted. I quit a job that was deeply unsatisfying and enrolled myself in graduate school so that I could do something that contributed to this world. That is my personal truth. It seems so ridiculous for someone to apologize to me for something that made me a better person, got my life back on track, and allowed me to live more clearly and authentically. I hope after reading this book you will feel the same.

No one is going to
understand YOUR
disease, and you can't
expect them to.

The truth of the matter is that if you do not personally have diabetes, you probably have no idea what it actually means. I bet you could not find two people in the room you are in right now that can accurately describe the disease or tell you the difference between Type 1 and Type 2. Until you are blindsided with diabetes or have a loved one with diabetes, you simply have no interest in knowing. It's something that happens to other people. To the average person, it seems scary, tedious, and life-threatening. I won't lie—it can be all of those things, but it does not have to come to that. However, I am not here to explain the medical component of diabetes. Whether you have Type 1 or Type 2, it is vital to understand how diabetes works biologically within your body and to seek out a qualified professional to aid you in your understanding of it.

I am writing all of this in order to address the emotional tsunami that comes along with your diagnosis and its inherent potential. I was diagnosed with Type 1 diabetes at the age of 39 and was completely unprepared for it. My emotions swung from utter shock to denial to anger and desperation. It just couldn't be! I was 5'10" and 140 pounds—the picture of health. How on earth could this be happening? How did I go from Happy Hour without a care in the world to holding a syringe in my hand with the working end pointed at my own soft abdomen? Could I possibly do this even once, much more for the rest of my life? I began to feel dizzy as I envisioned scurrying off to the bathroom to administer my shots, never enjoying another one of my mom's chocolate chip cookies (that taste like a reason to live), having to deal with millions of fingersticks, dialysis, blindness, numb hands and feet, amputations...aaaaggghhhhh!!! I was overwhelmed!

Before I go further, I understand that not everyone is going to sit on the ground and cry because they receive a diagnosis of diabetes. I've met individuals who grew up watching a parent manage diabetes and did not react as if it were a tragedy at all when they developed it themselves. Also, sometimes a person's reaction to a difficult or shocking event is to simply not react at all. Whatever the case may be, give yourself time to understand and process what has occurred so that you can stay connected to your emotions. This will help you make good decisions.

When I was first diagnosed, all I could do was cry—and I am *not* a crier. I cried in my doctor's office, and I cried when he sent me to the emergency room. I cried when I got home; I cried on the way to the specialist's office; and I cried all the way back home. I cried, cried, cried! I had no one to address my feelings with. I desperately needed for someone to grab me by both shoulders and say, "I have it, and you have it, and I'll help you."

I wish I could say everything will be okay for you, but I don't know that because I don't know you or how you are managing your disease. I can, however, show you the ropes because I have been there. I am there.

When I say I had no one to address my feelings with, I want to explain that I did have friends and family who were providing support, but none of them had diabetes. They could empathize with me, but they had no real understanding of the disease or the journey through it. This is different from a person I encountered in one of my support groups who chose to keep her disease to herself. She had just moved to the area and had one friend. She did not share with her friend or even tell her mom for more than a year. Even then, she was reluctant to do so. It took her two years to find her way to a support group, which was basically her first opportunity to discuss her feelings. If you are a private person and would like to receive support anonymously, online forums such as TuDiabetes offer you the opportunity to express yourself, ask questions, and forge friendships with other diabetics, and all that can be accomplished in the privacy of your own home. The important thing is to know you are not alone and there is a support system and connection available to suit your comfort level.

There are 25 million Americans with diabetes, and roughly six million do not even know it. You apparently do, so let's get on with it. The lid needs to be blown off the tidy box of myths surrounding diabetes, which is placed neatly out of sight. We as a society need a new vocabulary for communicating with people who have a disease. In our culture, we find it repugnant to face the truth of it, and this needs to stop. You are not "done for," and you hopefully have lots of living left to do. With some adjustments, you can accomplish anything anyone else can.

> ...understanding is more likely achieved with a level head.

When I was first diagnosed, I knew nothing about the disease. My dad drove me to the bookstore, and we loaded up on knowledge. I even bought *Diabetes for Dummies* and cookbooks. Buying the cookbooks was truly hilarious as I did not know how to cook at all.

The first thing I realized is that all of the books say basically the same thing, so just buy one that looks comprehensive and try not to overload yourself. You have a lot going on and not a lot of time, at this point, for leisure reading. If you are anything like I was, I just thought I couldn't eat sugar anymore. I encourage you to enter into the education phase of this journey with an open mind. Approach it with the mindset of "I know nothing, so anything I read or experience is of value." There is a lot of misinformation out there, so be sure to collaborate with your medical professionals. Slow down and breathe—understanding is more likely achieved with a level head.

> ...focus on the concern that is shown instead of the words that are said and just say thank you.

As I stated earlier, everyone will feel very sorry for you and will apologize and have very sad looks on their faces. It's best to focus on yourself right now instead of trying to take on pity. Remember, they probably have no idea what the disease really is. This is not the end of the world. In fact, it's the beginning of a healthier life if you choose it to be. Try to focus on the concern that is shown instead of the words that are said and just say thank you. Your loved ones will inevitably want to help so badly, but they do not know what you need, so just be real and open and allow them to have reactions, too. In times of uncertainty, people sometimes say very weird things, and they also tend to overreact. You are still trying to figure out which end is up yourself, so do not take any information as accurate from someone who is not a trained professional or physician. You should also be discerning with the information given to you by a physician. If it doesn't feel right, ask another doctor. Collaboration is always a good idea. Diabetes is very much like a fingerprint. There are similar components, of course, but the more you learn about the disease, the more you realize, like life, your diabetes is yours alone.

I am a very Type A person, and I remember wanting a formula that worked every time so that I could keep a steady 100 blood glucose level (BGL). Well, that's not even possible for someone without diabetes! When the doctor would tell me things like, "Just adjust it by one to two units and see what happens. You know, play with it." PLAY WITH IT??? That just made me cringe and added to my stress level—which you will learn directly affects your ability to manage your diabetes. I was very extreme and was prepared to eat the same thing every day so that I could control my sugar to a "T" without fail. I quit drinking alcohol altogether and my social life died right before my eyes. It was all way too much all at one time.

As far as showing emotion and needing support, please try to allow others to at least console you. I would melt behind closed doors so no one could see me fall apart, and then I would get mad when I didn't get sympathy. If you need a hug, an acknowledgment, or even a sympathetic ear, it's okay to ask for it.

In my experience, not only did no one understand my diabetes, they did not dive in with me to better educate themselves. I felt like I was on a deserted island. People can pay attention to diabetes for about 30 to 60 seconds before their eyes glaze over, so I will give you what I refer to as an "elevator speech" later in the book. It will give you a 30-second description of diabetes that anyone can understand. My own mother only read the first few pages of one of the books on diabetes that I bought. Why on earth would I have expected my friends to engage in this edification with me?

Remember, diabetes is something that "happens to someone else." It is amazing how quickly life resumes after something traumatic happens. Nothing that ever happens to you will be as important to someone else as it is to you. When the people around me horrifically resumed their lives, I began to feel a chasm grow. Their lives went on, and mine was forever changed. I pouted and secretly plotted not to be there for them either. But what I realized, with time, was that I *did* need them, and my health was my responsibility.

It is just simply human to sometimes be reduced to a creature in pain. Diabetes will peel it all away from you. You can only ignore it for so long because even if you try to live your life as you once did … it doesn't work. You don't react to food or drink the same way. Your body responds differently to exercise. It affects your sleep, your moods, your eyesight, your reality. It is a complete and total game changer.

When I got the diagnosis, I was scared. I was mad. I was resentful and needy at the same time. It broke me wide open. I had no idea what to do with the information or even what to think about it. I had no idea a whole new life was waiting for me to catch up.

Even if you think you have the situation under control and you do not feel emotionally assaulted by your diagnosis, make an appointment with a counselor that specializes in this sort of thing and see them a few times before you start with the support group option. You will be stronger and better able to handle a public appearance. The counselor that's right for you should have a wealth of resources and information for you about support groups. Your local Juvenile Diabetes Research Foundation will also be a tremendous resource for support. This can apply to the newly diagnosed as well as someone who has been trying to manage diabetes for a number of years. I say this because the longer you have the disease, the more desensitized you become to the consequences. Basically, you get used to bending the rules and letting bad decisions slide until you find yourself with an A1C level (average blood sugar) that reflects poor control. Seeking a counselor that specializes in diabetes can help you get back on track and can be a good part of disease management throughout your lifetime. Think of it as a tune-up for your mind and your management.

Reclaim calm.

Okay, so a bomb has gone off in your life. There will be phases you will go through to achieve acceptance; but for now, try to find a way to calm yourself. I remember that feeling of not believing what was happening. It takes a while to fully wrap your mind around the reality of the situation, so just deal with something tangible right now. It is only human to be blown away by this diagnosis.

After receiving my diagnosis, I remember finding a sliver of peace, and then BAM, there was the word "DIABETES" in red blinking lights in my mind's eye that would instantly dump a new batch of adrenaline into my stomach and send me reeling for hours. Mentally, it was like I was strolling down a peaceful sidewalk when all of a sudden, a rabid dog charged at me from the bushes and terrified me. This is what happens when you lack knowledge and your imagination takes over.

Your state of mind is something you can focus on and do something about. Try to stay in the moment and realize you are still here. Diabetes may change a lot of things about your life, but your reactions and your thoughts still belong to you. You choose the emotional path you want to take, but to be shocked and dismayed is understandable. Allow yourself that, but keep in mind it is not advancing the ball in any way. Whether you stay spun out for an hour or for the next year is one hundred percent your choice. Also keep in mind that it is everyone else's choice, too. The people in your life may actually have more trouble dealing with your diagnosis and for a longer period of time than you do. Do not allow this to impede your development. Respect them and their right to process what has happened however they choose to, but the show must go on for you and fairly quickly. You simply have too much to manage to allow for depression and denial. I believe these evil twins do more damage than the actual disease and left unattended can rob you of quality of life. Don't be lulled into a false sense of security just because you don't have Type 1 diabetes. A common myth is that Type 2 is not as bad as Type 1. Don't believe it—it does the same damage to your body as Type 1.

For myself, there was an initial insanity that I allowed to wash over me for about a week. I don't know how I made it through. That first week was a doozy for me with the hospital stay, diagnosis, and those first self-administered injections. They tried three different oral medications before determining insulin was necessary, and then I was on two different types of insulin. One type, I injected up to four times a day. The other was a once-a-day injection. I was a very busy sales executive with an even busier social calendar. How was this going to work? It is like my life exploded and all the pieces were suspended in the air around me.

> Don't be lulled into a false sense of security just because you don't have Type 1 diabetes. A common myth is that Type 2 is not as bad as Type 1. Don't believe it—it does the same damage to your body as Type 1.

I'm not going to sugarcoat it. Everything will and should stop for the time being. You need time and space and clarity to put it all back together in a different way that will work for you. If you have Type 2, you may be on pills rather than injections, but it still requires the same attention. There comes a time that you must depart from the entanglements in your life for your own sake. Sometimes a moment alone with yourself, possibly for the first time in your life, determines the rest of it.

Your diagnosis has brought you to one of these moments. You have the opportunity to be in the moment

with yourself and decide how you will move forward.
I know this may sound crazy to you, in the place you
are at the moment, but I for one am so grateful for the
opportunity of my moment. I was given a chance to
know myself and what I can truly do when called upon.
It was a hard blow; and I not only weathered it, but I
also used it to make myself better than ever before. I
would have been a weaker person without it. I don't
want to say I *needed* diabetes, but I can say I am eternally grateful for it. I couldn't see that in the beginning.
It took time and evolution and epiphany after epiphany
after epiphany. This disease brings a journey with it; and
like any journey, it brings a change in perspective that
you have the power to accept as positive or negative.
Every time I would realize my life was better than it
ever had been before, I could trace it back to having
diabetes. All roads of my current success lead back to
being diagnosed and the changes that came with it. I
have a richness about my life that I never had before. I
told a friend not too long ago that before I had diabetes,
I had a million people around me and felt I had nothing.
Now I have a handful of cherished people around me,
and I feel I have everything.

Another great thing to realize is you still have
options. When I was given the diagnosis, I felt power-
less, out of options or choices. It was a very long, con-
fusing, and painful road back to empowerment because
I did not have anyone to show me the ropes or tell me

> ...before I had diabetes, I had a million people around me and felt I had nothing. Now I have a handful of cherished people around me, and I feel I have everything.

that the best thing to do in this crazy time is to relax. Stress affects your body and your diabetes. "Find your center" would be the single most healthy and helpful advice someone could possibly give. A diagnosis of this magnitude is often like eating an elephant; you must take one small bite at a time.

It's essential to find a way to ground yourself. Meditation and focused breathing techniques are physical exercises that are used to calm the body and mind and can be very empowering and useful in a time like this. If you do not feel comfortable seeking out a meditation class or group in your area, there are plenty of podcasts and websites you can utilize in the comfort of your own home. There are even apps for smartphones and tablets that guide you through breathing techniques. Whatever you decide to try, just seek out some form of relaxation.

Jana

I sat dressed as a pumpkin, smiling and handing out Halloween treats at the carnival at the Children's Hospital. It broke my heart to see such young faces going through such health trials, but I only had a few hours to spare. I had to get home, shower, and change for a fashion event with my best friend at NorthPark Center that evening. I shoved my needles, tester, sugar pills, alcohol wipes, iPhone, and lip gloss into a clutch and went about my night, jealous of the champagne in everyone's hands, but smiling the entire time. I repeated my internal mantra that worse things had happened to better people, convincing myself of my emotional stability. The day before, I had been diagnosed as a Type 1 diabetic.

On October 28, 2009, I had walked into the doctor's office, anxious to figure out why I felt so terrible, and I walked out devastated and changed forever. I was 29 years old, and I was a newly diagnosed Type 1 diabetic. My first question to the doctor was, "I have a Halloween party this weekend. Can I drink?"

I decided a couple hours later it wasn't going to change my life. Two days later, I sat at a fashion show, hiding my pens in my clutch, eating carpaccio and drinking soda water because I didn't know how to process the math of blood sugar, carbs, and insulin. Two weeks later, I lost my job and sat in tears on the couch for two days. Everything changed. My social life, my diet, my relationship with my boyfriend, my pantry, the way my clothes fit, grocery shopping, my job—everything.

At the time, my ten-hour fasting blood sugar was 287, and my A1C was 12.1. I'm grateful I walked myself into the doctor's office and wasn't carried into the E.R. I'm grateful I had spent the previous summer working with a personal trainer and eating somewhat healthy. And I'm grateful (most of the time) that I was diagnosed with Type 1 diabetes.

I moved out of my apartment and in with my boyfriend of one year. After discussing the changes and what I was facing as my immediate future, he offered to stand by my side and hold my hand all the way through it. Six months later, my A1C was down to 6.8 and has been in that neighborhood ever since.

Because of my illness, I take better care of myself. I pay attention to what I eat. I'm able to counsel friends on nutrition and help those I love focus on their own health, even if it is just because they're scared to end up like me. No, you can't catch diabetes and you can't do anything to prevent my autoimmune Type 1 diabetes. But I can see it in their eyes that they're sad for me and glad for themselves. But I'm glad for me.

Since being diagnosed, I've taken more control of my life than I've ever had before and become closer to what I consider my support group of family and friends. My boyfriend and I opened a small boutique together, and now I'm in control of my everyday—when I take a break, how long I work, what snacks are in the mini-fridge in the back. Owning the business means no breaks, 60 hours a week, and lots of snacks instead of meals. But I am in control—not just of the store, but of my life. And I never would have taken the risk or felt the need to seize the day if I were never diagnosed.

I'm not alone. I recently joined a small study of newly diagnosed adult onset Type 1 diabetics. Each person in the group made a life-changing decision after coming to grips with his or her diagnosis. It's different for each of us, but it spurred each of us to, I guess you could say, pursue our dreams, follow our destinies, or honestly just work our butts off to get what we want out of life. If you let it, it instills a sort of determination once you embrace your new life and take control of your every day.

Most days I am more grateful than not about my diagnosis. I still get angry. I still get sad. It's very hard. But mostly I'm happy for the person I've become and the life I was driven to lead. I'm happy for the quality in my life I didn't even know I was missing before. And I'm so blessed to be able to lean on such an amazing support group I was only acquainted with emotionally before that day in 2009. On October 28, 2013, my boyfriend and I will be together five years, four of which I've been a diabetic. And I don't know at this point that either of us would want to go back.

Establish what you think about what has happened to you.

Albert Ellis, a famous psychologist who was a pioneer in using logic to resolve emotional issues, once said, "It isn't what has happened to you that is the cause of emotional pain. It is what you think about what has happened to you." In other words, it is your thought process about how diabetes is going to affect you that dictates whether your diagnosis is a good thing or a bad thing. Do you see this as a loss or a gain? Are you somewhere in the middle? Once you have diabetes and have reclaimed a calm mindset, it is your choice to look at your situation as a challenge, an opportunity, a lesson, or, perhaps, a wake up call.

I had a distant family member who had diabetes and was well into his 80s when I was diagnosed. He had lost a kidney when he was a child and had acquired diabetes in late adulthood. He died of heart failure at age 87. His death could possibly have been related to his diabetes, but there are plenty of people who die of heart failure before 87 years of age who do not have diabetes. He had never had an amputation and lived a very normal life. He ate sweets and bread and managed his disease better at times and not so well at other times. He is the perfect example of someone who lived a full and happy life with diabetes. You will find as you emerge from the fog of your diagnosis there will be things that resonate with you, and this was one of those lifelines for me. It was one of those moments in the midst of incredible intensity where reason finds its way into complete darkness like a lone ray of light—a moment where one simply sits up straight and says, "Oh. Yeah, this might not be so bad."

There are plenty of stories on either side of good or evil with diabetes. For every good story, there is a horrifyingly sad one. At first, you will want to hear it all, and you plug in, voraciously soaking every bit of information up like a sponge.

Quickly, for me, it became noise that I chose to tune out because most of what worked for someone else did not seem to apply to MY diabetes. Someone else's management is not specific to your disease and will not work as efficiently as really digging in and knowing what works for you individually. Now, I don't mind talking with someone and finding little similarities or sharing helpful information, but to try to apply someone else's formula to my own life is just a colossal waste of time.

There are so many similarities between how you manage your diabetes and how you live your life, and I will get to this in a following chapter; but when it comes to reaching out to others, your time would be better spent focusing on yourself and finding out what works for you. For the most part, others will follow your lead as far as how to think about you and your diabetes. If you are not careful, it can spill over into every area of your life.

This is what my mom and I primarily discussed. We talked about what I had for breakfast, lunch, and dinner; what my blood glucose level (BGL) was before each meal; and what they were two hours after. She would ask what my levels were when I woke up and when I went to bed. I appreciated it in the beginning because it helped me to not feel so alone. However, with the passage of time, levels will be all over the place; and when I would tell her numbers that were not so good, I felt as if I were reporting bad grades. In that space between the question and the response, I began to feel the urge to lie in order to evade—not good.

This disease is your responsibility—good, bad, or indifferent. Setting yourself up to lie about it or to evade the truth of it—to approach it with denial in any way— is just not healthy. Six years later, my parents still ask me periodically how things are going, but for the most part, they trust that I take care of myself. We can go an entire visit without even bringing it up.

You have the power to invite those around you to pity you or see you as a responsible adult who possesses the strength and grace to handle what life throws you. What you choose can actually increase your personal power. It's up to you. There is a theory that we grow by acquiring skills. If we operate under this theory, what we need to do to grow beyond the shock and dismay of the diabetes diagnosis is to acquire skills that make us feel more confident and empowered. This will be your key to sanity and peace.

> The point is the disease progresses, and damage continues even when there are no outward signs.

On the other hand, I have seen individuals use their disease as a way to promote themselves and, in the process, make it a way bigger deal than it actually is. They tell everyone around them they are diabetic. They garner sympathy and use it as an excuse to stay home, to not socialize, to gain weight, to get special treatment, or to get attention. I went to one support group that met at a greasy hamburger place, and everyone sat around and laughed about episodes of low blood sugar. It wasn't exactly what I was looking for. I am all for seeing the humor in life, even things on the darker side, but laughing about losing consciousness just isn't one of them.

Beware of people who seem to be able to circumvent the system with no consequences. This could come in the form of bragging about how high or low their blood sugar levels have been or just an overall flippant attitude about their management. The truth of the matter is that they probably do have consequences—just not on the surface. It reminds me of the cool kids in high school when they talked about skipping school. I really wanted to be cool and ditch, too, but the reality was the one time I did, they called my mom, I got paddled in front of her, and I had to do my schoolwork anyway. How's that for cool? The point is the disease progresses, and damage continues even when there are no outward signs.

If you do it right, you get to do it less.

All I could think about when I received my diagnosis was the amount of time I would be investing in the maintenance of this disease. There is so much coming at you at once, and it is very hard to focus on the bigger picture in the first few minutes, hours, and days of diagnosis. What I did not understand was that life would smooth out. I would learn how to work my meter. I would learn how food, exercise, and illness would affect me in time.

I urge you to not get overwhelmed in the moment. The advice I would give is to pick one thing and focus your energy on mastering that one thing. For me, it was purchasing a blood glucose monitor at the drug store and learning how to check my blood sugar. This will put you in the game and will allow you to gain some control immediately. Your blood glucose monitor is your first line of defense and will always put your hands on the steering wheel of your disease. No matter where you are, keep it with you. It is the only way you know where you are in the beginning because your body is adjusting so much. You cannot test too much. If you feel odd, check your sugar. If you are experiencing emotions that are not in line with what is happening around you, check your sugar. If your body temperature is out of line, check your sugar. Until you begin to calm down and adjust to the insulin or medication, keep your monitor with you like a baby keeps a blanket.

With time, things become instinctual, but I still test more on some days than others. It takes seconds to test and seconds to correct, and then you can move right on with life. I recorded the actual amount of time it took me to manage my diabetes on a typical day, which included testing, determining the amount of insulin needed for a specific meal, and administering a shot. It was right under 15 minutes.

I don't want my tombstone to say, "She should've checked her sugar." I want mine to say, "Here lies the longest living human in history!"

I do not want to make it sound like I have ever completely forgotten about my disease. In the case of any physical change, my diabetes is always what I investigate first. However, there are large amounts of time during the day that I live without that being my every waking thought. I am not taking away from the seriousness of this disease, but I will tell you with time and practice and self-awareness, it will get easier.

> One of the nurses told me that I had been blessed with a chronic illness because now I had a reason to be in the best health of my life.

When I think about not taking care of my disease and the repercussions of such behavior, I look at the amount of time that a hospital stay or repeated trips to various doctors to treat what neglect can cause would take. If we look at the extreme of what neglect can do, it can rob you of years of your life. It makes sense to simply take care of myself. I don't want my tombstone to say, "She should've checked her sugar." I want mine to say, "Here lies the longest living human in history!" I understand through my own experience that the mere mention of five shots a day sounds like there would hardly be room for bathroom breaks in between, but the reality is a shot just takes a few moments of attention. If you do not take insulin, it's even less.

One of the nurses told me that I had been blessed with a chronic illness because now I had a reason to be in the best health of my life. She was right. If this hadn't happened to me, I would still be drinking like a fish, eating takeout food three times a day, and getting little to no sleep. It made me realize that living the way you should in a responsible manner usually allows for a much more enjoyable experience and an opportunity for more than you had hoped for out of your life. It is an odd sensation to realize the thing you feared is really your chance at metamorphic growth.

Patrick

When I was diagnosed at the age of 20, I tried to convince myself that it was a shock and it was unexpected. In reality, it had always been in the back of my mind given the high rate of Type 1 diabetes in my family. My predisposition and prior experience with the disease proved to be a curse and a gift. Although the diagnosis was definitely not easy to hear and handle, having people in my life who had been through exactly what I was dealing with made a world of difference.

I watched my father handle this disease for two decades before it was my turn to do the same. It was as if I had been preparing my whole life for it. My family had always been very open about my father's condition, and we all shared in the responsibility of eating well, managing our health, and watching out for each other. With my family's support, I was back at school a week after my diagnosis. I was back at work two weeks later, and my life was back to "normal" within a few weeks—not to say that this disease is anything but complicated.

Not only was I lucky enough to have a network of fantastic diabetics to rely on, but I also had amazing friends to help me deal with the social and the psychological impacts of being diagnosed with Type 1 diabetes as a college student. They were supportive and caring, but they didn't let me get away with anything. They asked questions about my health, my disease, and how I treated it. They wanted to educate themselves to support me. They didn't let me feel bad for myself because they definitely weren't going to pity me. They knew, maybe naively, that this wasn't going to stop me or change me.

Everyone in my life helped me get the tools, the knowledge, and the right attitude to live with this diagnosis and manage it. My endocrinologist put it beautifully the first day we met when she said, "Be prepared to spend the rest of your life educating people about your disease." This truly is your disease, and you have to become your own expert. It is entirely manageable and not a death sentence if you take charge of your health, life, and wellbeing. There are days where things will go haywire and you will feel like things are out of control, but don't focus on reacting to the symptoms; focus on dealing with the cause. No one will ever care about your own health as much as you do. Sometimes, you need to be a bit selfish, live for yourself, and do whatever it takes to be a happy person living with diabetes. Be prepared to spend the rest of your life educating yourself, constantly learning, and balancing your life.

How you manage your life is a good indicator of how you will manage your disease.

believed diabetes was going to ruin the life I was currently living, and it did. I had been in medical insurance sales for about 11 years at that time. I was a Type A, driven person who had very little patience or tolerance. In an industry that encouraged relationship building in an intensely competitive environment, drinking was not only encouraged, but at times it was required and a measure of your commitment to the team. I lived life at warp speed and traveled constantly for business, for pleasure, and sometimes for both. I had a million friends who were constantly around me. Everyone wanted a piece of me because I was always the first one to Happy Hour and the last one to leave. I was always game and always a good time. I had tried to stop drinking previously and realized that translated to long, boring nights at home alone, so it was always back to the bars and the party.

I began having these heat surges that would turn the palms of my hands bright red. I could feel one coming on and would actually watch my hands turn red and then back to white. I would drink one bottle of water, a soft drink, or a sports drink right after another. I would drink two or three glasses of water before bed and fall asleep with my mouth as dry as a bone. I would have overwhelming hunger and practically eat like a ravenous dog at every meal. I decided to make an appointment with my family physician just to see if he had an opinion. I did not even have diabetes in my mind as a possibility. When I arrived at my doctor's office, he listened to my symptoms intently as I spewed them out as annoyances. I had a life to lead, and we needed to do something about whatever this was so I could get on with it. He checked my blood sugar, and it was so high the meter could not register it. I was immediately checked into the emergency room and the shock was indescribable.

I took a long, hard look at my life and realized immediately it was not going to accommodate my new diagnosis of diabetes. The two just could not coexist. If I took a rigid, impatient, bullying, and perfectionistic approach to managing diabetes, I would be incredibly hard on myself, which would lead to poor manage-ment and low self-esteem. Like many Type A personas, I tend to demand perfection from myself, and when this is not accomplished, I internalize it and begin beating myself up. When you beat yourself up, you are essentially saying you aren't good at whatever it is you are attempting. This sets you up for poor management and damages what is called your "locus of control." Locus of control basically describes the elements in your life that you believe are within your control. It is easier to abandon something you do not believe you are good at performing before you have given yourself a real shot at developing it.

So I had to overhaul myself. For me, this involved intense therapy in order to deal with emotional issues long buried with denial and heaping helpings of numbing self-medication. I self-medicated with alcohol, by overbooking myself with meetings and personal commitments, and with relationships and financial irresponsibility. Where in the world would diabetes fit into that scenario? It was definitely time for a change.

Denial is probably more dangerous than having any type of disease because it keeps you disconnected from reality. If you are in denial about anything in your life, it is infinitely more likely for you to be in some degree of denial about your disease. And even when you are acutely aware of the possibility of denial knocking you off track, with time it still snakes its way back into your management efforts. I still find myself doing the "insulin shuffle" in my mind. For instance, if a colleague brings cookies, my inner voice yells, "COOKIE!" just like Cookie Monster. I might start talking to myself about how I can just pick one up and eat it because I took a little too much insulin at lunch, and I'll just have one and be okay because I may go low later...blah, blah, blah. No. Reality is I need insulin for almost anything I eat. I certainly need it for a cookie. So, if I want one, I must take a shot. Period.

> If you are in denial about anything in your life, it is infinitely more likely for you to be in some degree of denial about your disease.

This is why it is great to be part of a support group. It can help you get back in the game of healthy diabetes management when you stray off the path, no matter which type you have. There are lots of different types of support groups. You can join an online social network. There are groups that meet for breakfast. There are groups that meet to discuss emotional aspects of the disease. Any group will do when you need to bring your management back into clear focus. Like Cesar Milan says about dogs: dogs are pack animals. He regularly brings a dog with a behavior problem into a pack of other dogs in order to correct the animal. I believe the same concept works for humans. Being part of a group gives you a chance to see how everyone else is doing it, thus rejuvenating your own efforts and getting you moving back in a positive direction. You do not have to attend religiously or even regularly. Go when you feel it is necessary or could possibly contribute to your management practices. Make sure it is a group that welcomes and encourages you whenever you do want to participate and does not badger you to attend or shame you when you do not. You are making space for your disease and practicing self-care when you make decisions that allow for a comfortable space for you and your needs. Keep in mind this type of behavior should not disrupt other emotionally healthy adults.

I am not into telling stories in order to shame or scare, but I had an experience in my childhood I would like to share. My best friend had a diabetic stepmother who did not manage her disease well. She was constantly having bouts of low blood sugar that resembled being drunk. She would have seizures and was regularly being driven to the hospital in an ambulance after being strapped down and babbling wildly, out of her mind. Sadly, she lost a leg and ultimately her life. She refused to manage her disease. She drank too much, ate whatever she wanted, and took either took too much insulin or not enough. Thankfully, managing diabetes does not have to be like that. The methods for testing blood sugar and delivering insulin have advanced so much since that time, but the decision to manage your health is still yours to make. With all the latest and greatest that traditional medicine has to offer, it still does not medicate for you. *You* have to do it.

It's encouraging to know that this is the best time in the history of mankind to be diagnosed with diabetes. My distant relative and my friend's stepmother are from generations who had no means of monitoring blood sugar, as testing strips and glucometers were not developed until the 1970s. The best one could do, at that time, was to use Ketone strips. By the time someone tested positive for Ketones in his or her urine, their blood sugar levels were already revved up into the danger zone. We now have convenient strips that plug into our personal monitors and allow us to instantly know what our level is anytime, anywhere. We have convenient pre-filled pens that are user friendly and fit in a pocket or a purse.

We have more advanced tools and more advanced information about diet and exercise in today's world. I encourage you to take advantage of these conveniences. Today's climate is also more accepting than ever before of acknowledging and dealing with emotional issues that are detrimental to healthy life functioning. It benefits you, your family, and everyone around you. I encourage you to incorporate this into your diabetes management as well.

Be open to your overall opinion changing about diabetes and what it means to you often.

nitially, with such little understanding of my disease, I felt the grim reaper's hot breath on the back of my neck. It was surreal, and I did not have the words to explain what was happening. It all became too real. It hurt me, and I felt sucker-punched. Diabetes—the unwelcome houseguest.

As time passed and I stabilized emotionally, I began to see it differently. Diabetes actually weeded out the relationships and connections in my life that were not healthy. I felt like it made my phone stop ringing, but then I asked myself what it was that I was no longer providing for my friends. Hours in a smoky bar? Evening after evening of commiserating girls' nights about the same old problems that, with alcohol, just become circular conversation? I wanted to move forward; and with the diagnosis, I got a big "Well get on with it!" from the universe.

It's hard to feel hostility toward something that has changed your life for the better—or at least provided the motivation! It sounds silly to attribute any cognitive ability to a disease. A disease isn't a person who can make decisions about someone's life. However, how you think about what the disease means to you and the effect it has on your life is all in the relationship that you build with it. We cannot change certain things in life, but we can find a way to live with just about anything. It is up to you to construct a personal relationship with the things that happen in your life, and diabetes is no different. Diabetes is not to blame. It is to respect."

> Diabetes is not to blame. It is to respect.

It has been six years for me, and I've watched all the tiny little pieces slowly come back together to form something completely different. I've learned so much. I've made totally different connections. I've grown spiritually and emotionally. I've gone to the outer parameters of who I am, and I've pulled it all back into center. Diabetes is not to blame. It is to respect.

I can also tell you that your age is a major contributing factor to how you perceive having diabetes. Children want to eat candy and eat birthday cake, and they most definitely don't want to appear different from their peers. This makes accepting diabetes difficult and resisting management easy. Young adults want to party and eat pizza at 3 a.m. They stay up late and have very little regularity in their lives. It's got to be annoying to manage diabetes in the middle of all the preparation they have to do for being a grown-up. But for more mature adults, it can be easier to moderate because we are slowing down and seeing the importance of good health. We no longer feel bulletproof, and managing our disease makes perfect sense and also gives a deep feeling of satisfaction.

I can only speak from the "more mature adult" point of view, but what diabetes means to me now is a world away from how I felt initially. I went from seeing my diagnosis as my body betraying me to now seeing it as what inspires me to make better choices. It keeps me on top of my game by challenging and confounding me. It is never the same thing every day, but it's always there. Shouldn't such a close relationship be positive?

Resistance works against your efforts.

guess I should first define what I mean by resistance, as resistance has a slightly different meaning for diabetics. The forms of resistance are sort of hidden from view in the beginning; but as time goes along, you will sense them creeping in like a fog. When I say resistance, I mean any behavior or emotion that reassures you that you do not have a disease when, in fact, you do. For example, when you begin to eat a cupcake, ask yourself, "Have I prepared myself for this?" If you have checked your blood sugar and taken the amount of insulin you need for a cupcake, then ENJOY! If you tell yourself something like, "I don't have my insulin with me at the moment, so I'll eat this and take a shot later," or if you are Type 2 and say, "I'll take an extra pill," you are resisting having diabetes.

Any form of denial in conjunction with diabetes can jeopardize your health, Type 2 included. There will be times, of course, that you fudge your blood sugar levels to your mom or a loved one, but you should make a pact with yourself right now that you will not fudge it to yourself. Where diabetes is concerned, you cannot rely on gut feelings, or what your numbers should be, or even how you will smooth this all out later with more insulin and eating right. You must deal in honesty and reality with yourself at all times. If you are about to do something dumb, admit to yourself that it is dumb; and if that does not deter you, at least you cannot blame the consequences on the disease. Having consequences from poor diabetes management is like having consequences for poor eating habits. It takes a while, but it eventually does show. It is very difficult to reverse the process—in the case of diabetes, the effects are usually irreversible. Diabetes plays for keeps. This is a disease of management, not offense and defense.

The urge to minimize a high blood sugar level is very seductive and alluring. The desire to rationalize it all out in your mind—that you will fix it at the next meal—is strong. These behaviors can become habits that lull you to sleep; and before you know it, you are cramming cupcakes in your mouth like a preteen at the mall with a fully functioning pancreas, all the while telling yourself, "I'll just take a few extra units or another pill next time I eat." This leads to chronic high blood sugar, and this does not even have to happen as a result of an extreme example like the one I just gave.

It can be from eating a banana or drinking a glass of milk. You may not think that, in the big picture, one hour here or three hours there of healthy blood sugar matters, but it absolutely does! All of those little hours add up to days, weeks, and years by the time your life is over. I used to laugh at my roommate in college who would get onto me for buying a brand name of canned green beans instead of a store brand for 20 cents less. 25 years later, she is talking about retirement, and I feel like I'm starting all over again! It all adds up, good or bad. Over time, the choices you make tell a story about you. What will your story be?

Any form of denial in conjunction with diabetes can jeopardize your health, Type 2 included.

Another form of resistance is not incorporating physical exercise into your daily life. It is a little tricky because your blood sugar needs to be high enough so as not to become too low during a workout. However, this should not deter you from a 30-minute walk. There are professional athletes who have diabetes, and they do way more than just walk. You may hear a fellow diabetic say something like, "Well, if I have to eat a candy bar before I work out in order to not go low, the workout is meaningless!" This is faulty thinking because a candy bar is not the only option. A lot of behavior is fueled by what we tell ourselves; and if those thoughts are creating resistance for you, it may be time to start challenging some of your ideas. I saw a bumper sticker the other day that said, "Don't believe everything you think!"

"Don't believe everything you think!"

Patricia,

I have always been a healthy person in the sense that I did not have any ailments or allergies nor had I ever had any serious medical conditions...until the unexpected occurred. It triggered three years ago when I had been working long hours, going out partying, and traveling like crazy. My schedule was hectic, and I was extremely stressed. In addition to my chaos, I was feeling constantly exhausted, hungry, and thirsty. I thought it was due to the busy lifestyle I was living. Unbeknownst to me, I was living with diabetes and did not know it. Not only did I not know it but would have never guessed that I had a condition that would change my life entirely. During those stressful times, my body was in survival mode until, one day, I collapsed and was admitted into the emergency room with diabetic ketoacidosis. I was placed in an intensive care room where they would deliver the news. I had Type 1 diabetes.

My initial reaction to my diagnosis was disbelief. I thought the doctors made a mistake because I have never had any medical issues. Then reality set in, and I realized I had to change my whole lifestyle because of this condition. I was terrified that I had experienced such a dramatic episode and was trying to wrap my mind around the idea that I had to rely on insulin for survival. I had to monitor my eating, stop smoking cigarettes, and avoid drinking alcohol. My social and work life revolved around eating out and having drinks with customers and friends, and I had been a smoker for over ten years. The changes were imperative for my wellbeing. So, with a blink of an eye, I stopped my bad habits and started my journey cultivating good ones. Little did I know it would change my entire world. When I was at work, I was no longer going out to eat. Instead, I brought my lunch, which distanced me from my coworkers.

It was the same situation with my friends. I was no longer going out to bars to drink and smoke or dining out, so I was no longer included in the outings. At a time when I needed so much support, I found it was quickly slipping away because I no longer participated in the same activities. Initially, I could not understand how people I have known for years and shared so many great experiences with were becoming so distant, but eventually I came to terms with the idea that I had to move forward with my condition. I figured those who remained in my life would support me on my path and those who strayed were not people I wanted in my life going forward. It was a wake up call that I used to push myself to become stronger and better as well as an advocate for my own wellbeing. I became active, joining different programs to become more educated and involved in the diabetes community. Also, I participated in a variety of exercise programs and explored different activities that I felt I would enjoy. Eventually, I started to meet new people and found my own rhythm with my condition. I tried different activities, discovered new eating habits, and learned different exercise techniques. Moreover, I realized I reinvented my life into a manner that is now more productive and rewarding. I feel better, think clearer, play harder, and enjoy life with a different perspective. I am extremely grateful that I have this condition. It saved my life. I do not take anything for granted and am now aware that life changes and one must change with it.

You must initially change
your behavior to feel
better emotionally and
then adjust your emotions
to sustain behavior
changes permanently.

We often make choices for emotional reasons. If you are not in touch with your
emotions, healthy decision making is difficult. When the body is under physical
stress, such as with pain or illness, the emotional system
is burdened. This can set the stage for poor decision
making. At the heart of successful diabetes management
is good decision making.

Initially, your head is going to be filled with a million
different things; but when you do begin to embrace the
concept of diabetes in your life and what this is going to
mean, you will begin to formulate a plan to take care of
yourself. For some, there may be a strong urge to ignore

or deny what is happening. I urge you to shake this off and adopt a more positive mindset in order to begin on the right foot. As I have been told, it is easier to start something than to stop something.

For others, this may be the first time in your life that you give self-care a thought. Some of you may be well-adjusted and are already taking time for yourself and considering your wellbeing, which will enable you to possibly take a diagnosis of diabetes in stride. I admire those of you in this situation because it is so refreshing for those of us who were dismayed by the diagnosis to see such an example. It is great to see those with positive attitudes reaching out and modeling behavior for those who are not so fortunate. But the good news is a positive attitude is attainable for us, too!

As stated above, emotions and making decisions go hand-in-hand. Like I've said before, diabetes is just as much of an emotional condition as it is a physical condition. If you had any dysfunction in your decision-making processes before, they will be magnified with diabetes.

Before I was diagnosed, I made poor decisions for my health. I felt as if I were bulletproof and did not look my age even though I was abusing my body. I could eat anything and drink anything and still look a good ten years younger than my actual age. I sped through my days at lightning speed, firmly believing that it would never catch up with me. But it did; and when it did, I had no idea how to make a good decision for myself. Does this sound familiar to anyone? It should. As a culture, we tend to value ourselves on how much we can weigh ourselves down with work, family, school, exercise, socializing, and more. I thought I could carry anything on my shoulders with ease and still function at a high level, but any dysfunction is a heavy load. Diabetes gave me an opportunity to slow down and say enough is enough.

When you disconnect from your feelings, you do not have a relationship with yourself any longer, and bad decisions are easy to make. When you know yourself, connecting to your emotions becomes easier. When you are connected to your emotions, you can make a clear decision that is in your own best interest. Denying or suppressing emotions in order to make a decision that is best for someone else hurts you. It does this because you are not factoring yourself into the process, and you deserve as much as anyone else. If you have issues that have not been dealt with, I believe you owe it to yourself to take this opportunity to address them now. You, your body, and your spirit deserve the chance to live, and you are going to need to put your best effort into life with diabetes moving forward. When you are able to think clearly, you can better make decisions regarding your health and the choices you make on your own behalf. Behavior and emotion are forever linked, so be sure you are overseeing the process. Remember that the choices you make today impact the quality of your life tomorrow.

I want to expand a bit on what is meant by self-care. It brings to mind the old Saturday Night Live skit with Stuart Smalley. He was this nerdy guy who sat in front of a mirror and said, "I'm good enough. I'm smart enough. And doggone it, people like me." These types of affirmations were the butt of many jokes in its day; however, times have evolved, and there are more effective ways of having a relationship with yourself. Self-care simply means that you acknowledge your existence and your worth by doing something for the sake of your own wellbeing.

Through my journey, I have come to appreciate meditation. It is a way to breathe deeply and calm myself. I acknowledge my need for peace, and I satisfy it by cultivating calm energy. I also enjoy reading, so I make time for that each day, even if it is for ten minutes at night before I fall asleep. I acknowledge the need I have to take my brain offline, so I satisfy it by reading a book that interests me which provides a temporary escape from the day's concerns. I have a wonderful relationship with my parents, and I make time to spend with them, whether it is to eat a meal or just sit and share our lives. This makes me happy. I acknowledge this need I have by also satisfying it with a visit to my childhood home. I tend to hold tension between my shoulder blades and in my neck and shoulders. I acknowledge that I have to manage my stress, and I satisfy it with a trip to the massage therapist.

The term "self-care" seems like this mystical process or something that is selfish, but it is really anything but selfish. Think of a close relationship you have with a friend. If your friend had a problem and called upon you for help, you would acknowledge your friend and help them as best you could. We rarely treat ourselves with the same amount of acknowledgement and attention. This is what self-care is all about. Acknowledge your needs and make time to satisfy them.

You will feel worse before you feel better.

I n the beginning, my sugar levels were very high. High blood sugar levels affect mental capabilities, mood, physical wellness, eyesight, and sleeping patterns among other things. The process of getting my blood sugar levels back into a normal range felt odd. I didn't feel right in my own skin, and my eyesight went blurry for about six months, requiring me to wear contacts for the first time in my life. I felt as if I were walking through a surreal dream.

As I have stated before, I also took this time to become a healthier person. In my case, I quit drinking alcohol as well as sugar-based sports drinks and sodas, so part of my experience included kicking the great American sugar addiction. The ways people invent to ingest sugar never ceases to amaze me. I was living a very high-carbohydrate lifestyle. Anytime I got in my car, I religiously whipped into a quick mart of some sort to get a drink and a snack, usually a candy bar or chips. After my diagnosis, I found myself whipping into the quick mart only to roam the aisles reading labels and scratching my head. It's a quick mart—they sell quick energy! They stock their shelves with what sells, and that does not include Atkins bars or low-carb anything. The selections are improving with time, I must say, thanks to the low-carb craze and public demand for healthier choices. However, I still struggle to find "zero" drinks that are suitable for me. Most times, I just defer to the water section and toss around the idea of requesting that the owner provide a better selection on the way to the register.

This is a whole new way of life for some people, and there are definite physical changes that take place, but I believe your mindset is the most important thing one can cultivate. It is what you will use to make all of your decisions—your health starts there. When I was growing up and did not have the right attitude, my dad would tell me, "You better get your mind right, girl." That saying applies to this journey. Get the mindset right, and the physical goals will follow.

I am not talking about rigid rules and depriving yourself of anything with sugar in it. I simply mean adjust for a new lifestyle so that you can be healthy and not destructive to your new situation. This makes sense and is rational and responsible for any diabetic. Responsibility does not have to be associated with strict rule-following or rigidity. I try to do what makes sense, and part of that is realizing I cannot cram six chocolate chip cookies down my throat without ramifications any longer. Now I take a shot and have two. It's a meeting in the middle of sorts, and I walk away just as satisfied.

But gradually other things started happening, too. Before, I had a water bottle practically surgically attached to my hand. I was never, ever without a bottle of water. I had an unquenchable thirst and drank water constantly. Every drink was like a deep gulp that I felt down in my bones. When I began taking insulin shots, I remember realizing that I no longer had a water bottle in my hand, in my purse, on my desk, and in my car. I did not feel thirsty anymore—it was wonderful! My eyes were lubricated, and my skin even became smoother. My body was processing differently, and it felt awesome. I told my friend that it was hard to complain when you felt so good. Diabetes seemed to moderate my entire life, and I am deeply pleased with all aspects. It allows me to overlook 95% of the mechanics of shot taking and finger pricking. Now, even when it hurts, I just blow it off. It only lasts a few seconds, and the gains are immeasurable. We are so very fortunate to have the advanced tools with which to manage our disease in today's world. It is mind-boggling to think that test strips were only invented in the 1970s.

You may be at any various stage of shock, dismay, or acceptance as you read this book. You may have been diagnosed a month ago, ten or more years ago, or today. Your life has definitely changed, I will give you that, but it is truly all in how you look at it. I think it helps to know that you are going to fit into life differently now. It is mind-blowing to have life shift like this, but doesn't life change all the time anyway? Diabetes can be a catalyst for good changes. This can be an adjusting period based on reality and fact as you build your arsenal with information and knowledge of yourself. It's a chance to get to know yourself better than you may ever have before. It has calmed me, and it has given me courage to act and not procrastinate. I hope they cure this disease tomorrow, but I will always appreciate the impact it has had upon my life.

Diabetes can be a catalyst for good changes.

Rick

My short diabetes story is this: I was born to a mother suffering from her second round of gestational diabetes. Shortly after my birth, she was diagnosed as Type 1. Growing up, like most kids, I was completely unaware of the issues the disease created. I remember going to see my mother in the ICU multiple times; but honestly, at the time, I could not tell you why. Because of my mother's diagnosis, I took part in a diabetes study. The outcome was a prediction that I would be diabetic by the time I was a teenager—great. I never let it bother me but always kept it in the back of my mind and continued on as a normal kid. I was diagnosed my sophomore year of high school at fifteen years old. I was "The Diabetic." At first, it was awkward taking shots, explaining things, hearing "I am sorry," but shortly, I owned it. In a weird way, the attention was funny. Sadly, my mother lost her daily battle a year and a half after I was diagnosed. She was the kind of mother, friend, and person who would jump as high as possible for you at the drop of a hat. The reality is that diabetics, at times, have to be selfish. You must give your body the attention it deserves, or it will come back and bite you. Now, twelve years later, I am still known as "The Diabetic." I carry around multiple "iPods" that assist in making my life easier. I graduated from college where I participated in Greek life. I play multiple sports and have even started a company and still maintain good control. Easy? No. But you will learn how to power through the frustrations. Most importantly, become your own advocate! Try not to get frustrated by the people (everyone) who do not have a clue about the disease. It's nearly impossible to truly explain the complications involved, the ups and downs, the shaking, the confusions, the having to go home to change pods, and so on. There are many "experts," but few really are true experts. Diabetes is not just black and white. There is a tremendous amount of GRAY! First, and the most difficult, you have to accept the fact of your diagnosis. Everyone's body is different, and just about everything you do can and will affect your diabetes. Secondly, learn as much as possible. Speak with and get to know the experts so as to build your own opinion and knowledge. Lastly, surround yourself with individuals who have some understanding of diabetes (YOU may have to teach them.) Sure enough, you will have issues so it is best to be around people who can help.

Dealing with ignorance, apathy, and insensitivity

"But you aren't fat."

"You don't look sick."

"It's like you don't even have diabetes."

"So you can't have sugar, right?"

"So why don't you just eat right and exercise and stop taking insulin?"

These are just a few of the comments that have been said to me over the last six years. Watching those around me deal with my disease has been most interesting.

I mentioned in an earlier chapter that people will be likely to say some strange things at the time of your diagnosis. My advice was to not take it in but rather focus more on the concern they are showing than what they are actually saying. The truth is when something that is perceived as unfortunate happens to someone else, most people just really don't know what to say. In our culture, we are conditioned to feel sorry for other people and make judgments about what is good and what is bad for someone else. I think it is also within our nature to think the worst at the immediate moment of change but then later, with time, gain perspective.

> "But you aren't fat." "You don't look sick." "It's like you don't even have diabetes." "So you can't have sugar, right?" "So why don't you just eat right and exercise and stop taking insulin?"

For me, I was horrified at first; but as time passed, I realized it was right in line with the goals I had long wanted to achieve for my personal health. I believed this diagnosis would floor anyone that received it and then realized after interacting with many diabetics, some take it in stride and are not emotionally affected about it in the least. To make judgments about someone else's life situation is presumptuous. I don't spend time wondering what other people think about my diabetes. I don't excuse myself to the restroom in order to check my blood sugar and administer a shot. I know people who do, and that is their choice, as they have their own reasons for doing so. I personally don't feel that I have anything to hide, and most people don't even realize I have given myself a shot before our meal has started. I want to state, however, that there is a difference in handling what you need to do and spreading your kit out on the table top and making a production out of your diabetes. That is not what I am suggesting. Within reason, taking the necessary steps to manage your diabetes is good self-care.

In the same way someone may say something inappropriate to you, others may say nothing at all. This could appear as though they do not care when, in actuality, they may care very much. There are many different ways to react to another person's private issues, and some people might consider questioning you about your diabetes an intrusion. If someone is generally a private person, they may extend the same courtesy to you as a gesture of respect. So before you conclude that someone in your life does not care, just ask them what they think about your diabetes.

Helplessness may be another reason for someone in your life not dealing well with, or what you may deem dealing "appropriately" with, your diabetes. Sometimes an individual will avoid a topic they find painful. I had a friend who wanted me to continue behaving as I always had, but that was no longer possible. Because of her fear of my diagnosis, I saw less and less of her until we no longer spoke at all. I discovered later that it was so upsetting for her that she just could not face it by spending time with me. Instead of feeling abandoned, I realized it was her way of coping.

We tend to insert ourselves into the processes of those around us in order to make sense of their actions, and the reality of the situation is the only process we are a part of, or that we really understand, is our own.

The way to deal with the comments and behaviors of those around you is to really know yourself. When you believe in yourself, no one can come into your space and tell you who you are. It is calming and liberating. You have diabetes no matter what anyone's opinion of you may be. In the spirit of self-care, develop a healthy and positive self-opinion and put it first.

Guidelines for family members: boundaries, boundaries, boundaries!

This is probably the most difficult topic to maneuver around because your loved ones want the best for you. Like most things in life, this is a personal challenge. No one should stand over you and remind you to take your blood sugar. However, in their defense, they are as new to this situation as you are, and the tendency to ask about your management may be the only option they believe available.

In the initial confusion, you and your support system may find yourselves being hyper-vigilant around your sugar levels and what you eat, how much insulin you take, or if you took your pill while at the same time being in a mad scramble to educate yourselves, but things will calm down. When they do, take the reins. If you are ready for family and friends to back off, let them know that you have appreciated the support they have given, and now you would like to begin managing it on your own. Assure them that if anything major happens, they will be notified. It is okay to appreciate their support and make the choice to now ask them to trust you to manage your disease. This is establishing a boundary—a limit that you set for yourself in order to comfortably interact with those around you.

A boundary is not a wall. It is healthy and fair to let others know what your expectations are, and it still allows for an exchange to take place. Healthy exchanges cannot take place if you put up a wall, and you and your loved one will grow weary of it. So be open with those around you regarding how you want to incorporate the management of your diabetes and begin to move forward. If they violate the boundary with incessant inquiries or hovering, they need to take responsibility for that behavior. Then it is about their behavior and has nothing to do with your diabetes. Also, if you do not develop a sense of personal responsibility and make the disease your own, it could possibly create an almost addict-like cycle of ask, receive answer, and relief. Therefore, it will be even tougher to establish your independence because you want to keep your loved ones in the loop. There is a lot of adjusting for everyone involved, and having a game plan right from the beginning will set expectations for behavior and will allow everyone to be responsible for themselves. With this being said, if you do not want others involved, you actually have to manage your diabetes!

> A boundary is not a wall. It is healthy and fair to let others know what your expectations are, and it still allows for an exchange to take place.

This brings me to a subject I hear more and more about. Invariably, when people find out I am diabetic, they always have a story about someone they know who also has diabetes. One version I am hearing with more frequency is how someone is using their diabetes to get attention. Look, I'm not going to sit here and say I have never used my diabetes as an excuse to get out of some uncomfortable social function before, but to misrepresent yourself on a regular basis is not healthy. It is easy to garner sympathy because the majority of the population does not understand diabetes one iota; and due to the involvement of needles and contraptions that make your fingers bleed, they want about as far away from it as they can get. But as a diabetic, you and I both know that it is very tolerable. Sometimes I cannot believe I actually gave myself a shot. I actually wonder if the needle made it under my skin, and I watched it go under my skin! Sometimes it sucks, but most times it does not. I merely want to suggest that you at least have a small amount of healthy shame when you act like a damsel in distress.

You've made a departure from the life you currently know. Make the new one your own!

The way you think and feel about your life and the way you plan it will all be altered by this event. For me, it was a mind-blower, and all I could focus on was what I could no longer do. I swam around in all the myths about diabetes, and it just sank me deeper. I am a task-oriented person who likes to work autonomously, so I really dove right into the research part of having diabetes. This helped focus my anxiety into something positive. Once I stabilized my health and found a rhythm, I took an inventory of my life. It was my responsibility to take the new me and plug that back into society, not the other way around. I think I sat by passively and watched how others handled me, and then I realized the people in my life were looking to follow MY lead. Everyone has their own journey in life, and you are responsible for yours. It was never clearer to me than at that moment in time.

I want you to know that, if you are experiencing some of the same emotions, it gets better. Let some time pass, and perspective will come with it. Nothing is more cleansing emotionally as when something puts you on the ropes. It's an opportunity—a chance to move past obstacles that may possibly have kept you inert for years. It moved me past "I need alcohol for a social life," and "I can't go back to school and give up my comfortable salary," and landed me in a whole new place of clarity, strength, and personal empowerment.

> Diabetes puts your attitude in the Here and Now.

Diabetes is by far not the worst thing that could happen. In fact, it gives you the chance to live the life you always wanted to live and kept putting off for one reason or another. Diabetes puts your attitude in the Here and Now. It deepened me spiritually. It allowed me to be patient with myself. It weeded out the riff raff from my support system, and what remains is real and reliable.

Even though diabetes can be one of the best things to happen to your life, please be prepared for the people you believed would take a bullet for you to leave. I am not saying they will, but they might. It is absolutely heartbreaking, but keep in mind that people are entitled to their reactions. Whether they leave because the mechanics of taking shots bothers them, the sight of blood on your finger bothers them, not being able to help you bothers them, having to be sober is not comfortable for them, or whatever the reason may be, allow them to do it and stay on track with your journey and your tasks of being healthy. Find a good support group and a good therapist. Allow people who are qualified to support you to fill in the gaps. I know it feels as if you are losing parts of yourself; but with a slight shift in thinking, you may see that you are really more in control of how your life moves forward. You may find your decision making is clearer and rooted in a belief in yourself and not the pleasing of others.

In my observation, diabetes tends to ignite the broken things within you such as emotional problems, immaturity, and codependency. It uncovers things that need your attention such as the inability to meet your personal needs and placing the needs of others before your own. It also fuels wonderful things within you such as bravery, independence, and self-care. It is amazing how this disease gives you the opportunity to live life to the fullest or expedite the destruction of it. It's like a higher power says, "Okay, here it is! It's your choice, but we're about to get to it in a big hurry. So make up your mind which way this party is going to go!"

I conducted a diabetes support group and learned a tremendous amount from the wonderful people who attended religiously and poured their hearts into it. One of the things that reaffirmed what I learned before was that not all people experience an emotional crisis upon diagnosis. This was amazing to me because of my own personal experience of emotional devastation. But it helped me to realize some people roll with the punches of life and merely need more information.

Also, for those who do not roll with it so easily, there are varying degrees of shock. Some experienced an initial shock and made minor adjustments in their lifestyle and moved right on. Others were still in a bit of a quagmire. No matter where they were on the scale, getting together with like-minded others satisfied something deep within each of them and was a moving experience. I asked them to draw a picture of what diabetes means to them, and the descriptors used across the board were opportunity and courage to reach for their dreams. I think it gives you a wake-up call that this life is finite and you need to get a move on with what you want to get accomplished here today, not tomorrow. The attitudes and feelings you have right now will shift.

With time, you will begin to see how diabetes works on your life, and, in my experience, it has been a great teacher for whom I have much respect. Again, diabetes brings out the true YOU. I can look back on my life and see that it fits perfectly with how I approach complex problems. I went through shock, then I felt the constricting claustrophobia of not being able to change it, then I moved on to trying to understand it, and then in the end, when I realized it was here to stay, I began to make friends with diabetes and established a respect for the disease.

For a lot of people, they never leave the constricting claustrophobia stage, and bad decisions ensue. That is one reason why I wrote this book. We come to crossroads in our lives that require something of us. If you had trouble choosing a direction before diabetes, can you imagine how difficult it would be to arrive with this complicated disease on your back? I did not know who I was before I got diabetes. I can tell you now I do, and it is the most rewarding thing I enjoy on a daily basis.

Knowledge and time are your best friends right now. Find a good physician. Go through fifteen if you have to. Never settle until you find a compatible physician who understands you and what your needs are. I do not know if this has been for my own good at times in my life, but I am always cross-referencing information given to me with my personal truth. If I do not feel confident in what my doctor is telling me, I may feel they are not plugged into what I am trying to tell them or I just may not be getting my needs met with their style of health care. Whatever the case may be, find a physician who works for you. Also, like I've said before, local support groups are always a good source of information. I did not exactly relate to everyone I met, but it gave me an opportunity to gather knowledge and advice regarding physicians in the community and the experiences others had with them without having to waste time and money making an appointment.

It is my sincere hope that I am giving you options and a wider view into the future with sufficient knowledge about the emotional field that surrounds the already dynamic disease of diabetes. Knowledge is liberating and empowering and will help you get a handle on your situation. This will help pave the way for more tolerance in the relationship you build with your disease. A happy and healthy life with diabetes is possible.

Elevator Speech

What is Diabetes?

Insulin is a hormone that is created in the pancreas by something called Beta cells. When you eat food, it is converted to sugar, which your cells burn as fuel. For this to happen, the sugar has to find its way into the cell. Think of insulin as the doorman to the cell. When your cells need sugar, insulin opens the door and lets the sugar enter the cell from the bloodstream. If there is no doorman, no sugar can get into the cell. Therefore, the sugar is just free floating in your bloodstream. The sugar are like little crystals that are sharp, and this does damage to your vascular system, your nervous system, your eyes, your kidneys, and your heart because it shreds as it flows through your body, which is why it is so important to control the blood sugar as a diabetic.

The Difference between Type 1 and Type 2

When the Beta cells malfunction and no longer produce insulin, you have Type 1 diabetes. This condition creates a dependence on insulin that must be replaced with daily injections of insulin.

Type 2 is when, for many different reasons, your body becomes resistant to the insulin your pancreas is still able to produce. Because the Beta cells are still functioning and producing insulin for the body, many times Type 2 can be treated with oral medications. However, it is not uncommon for Type 2s to also be on some form of an insulin injection as well.

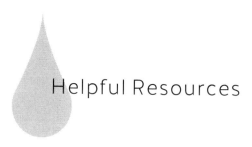

Helpful Resources

American Diabetes Association, www.diabetes.org
Juvenile Diabetes Research Foundation, www.jdrf.org
Tu Diabetes, www.tudiabetes.org

Meditation /Breathing Classes:
Search Google to find classes in your area. Search for podcast meditations on iTunes.

Smartphone Apps:
Search for these on the internet or through the App Store. Since everyone's needs are different there are no particular ones advocated.

Other Searches:
- Doctors—In my experience, it is a good thing to get involved in JDRF in your area and begin speaking with other diabetics in order to get

feedback about doctors in your area. There is no website that will give you honest feedback on a doctors wait time, sense of humor (or lack of one), ability to connect with you, or their afterhours accessibility. It is trial and error and the sooner you get involved with other diabetics in your community the more you will know.

- Therapists—The same applies here. There is no website that will give you the information you need in order to make an intelligent selection. Many are listed, but the best approach is to contact your local JDRF or ADA for resources in your area.

- Support Groups—You can contact your local JDRF or ADA for resources in your area.

Tanya

Kelley recently received one more letter from a fellow diabetic and felt it was important for her readers.

I was diagnosed with type 1 diabetes (T1D) when I was nine—39 years ago. I was fortunate and my mom took me to the doctor with very few symptoms, so I didn't have the terrible DKA (diabetic ketoacidosis) or life threatening situation that happens to so many people as they get diagnosed.

One of the most amazing things about this disease is how much progress has been made, and continues to be made related to care and approaching a cure! When I was first diagnosed, the only way to determine my sugar level at home was with a urine test. It involved voiding my bladder an hour prior to eating then drinking a glass of water, urinating right before meal time, and running this test with drops of urine in a test tube. I would visually match the color the solution turned to a chart and determine my level within a 50-point range. And THAT was hour old information since it was already in my urine, but it was the best we had.

My first take home blood sugar meter was about the size and weight of a brick and took somewhere between 3–5 minutes and a very large blood sample. But it was so much better than a urine test, I was happy. At that time there wasn't even such a thing as carb-counting or taking a ratio of insulin. Now the machines, technology and research we have are amazing! The Continuous Glucose Monitor (CGM) pretty much changed my life!

And research has us really close to some major, life-changing advancements in our near future. For example: smart insulin (one shot a day with nearly perfect blood sugars), encapsulation (protected beta cells that would be pretty much be a cure for 18-24 months) and an artificial pancreas (a pump and CGM that talk to each other and take the guesswork out of the equation). All super exciting!

Most of the time, I'm optimistic about the progress for this disease. But I certainly also get frustrated, angry, and depressed at times. I found for me that one way I can let out some of that negativity is through doing art about how I feel about all this and the messages I tell myself. I know that having a group of friends that are also living with T1D is another HUGE help. I get so much validation and commiseration from other adults living with T1D. And I'm sure there are other positive ways people have chosen to cope with this diagnosis.

My advice to other diabetics: always have sugar with you, and look for the positives in this situation. For example, I bet you know way more about your body than most folks, and can count carbs with the best of them! Good luck!